Your Amazing Itty Bitty™ True Healing Book

15 Ways to Approach Your Best Health

Angela Kung, L.Ac.

Published by Itty Bitty™ Publishing
A subsidiary of S & P Productions, Inc.

Printed in the United States of America

Itty Bitty Publishing
311 Main Street, Suite D
El Segundo, CA 90245
(310) 640-8885

ISBN: 978-0-9996519-5-7

This book is for educational purposes only. Nothing should be taken as medical or mental health advice, diagnosis or treatment. Always check with your doctor before changing your diet, altering your sleep habits or starting a new fitness routine.

Dedication

This book is dedicated to my mother, who has been a spiritual guide and angel to me in life and even more so since her passing. I had the privilege of holding her hand and being with her at her last breath, a fated experience that changed me. Helping her cross over and having her help me now in so many ways, including the knowledge that she was with me as I wrote this book, shows that love knows no bounds. We need not fear or feel abandoned by our loved ones who cross over. Thank you, Mom, for your undying love. I cherish the thought of being with you again someday. I feel you, I know you're there, and I love you.

This book is also dedicated to all those seeking true healing. You are not alone; God sees you, knows you, and will help you. Pray, meditate, and ask for help because miracles do exist. Love from the other side is so powerful that once you believe it, have faith in it, and act upon your intuitive promptings, you too can have the life you've always wanted. I'm living proof of that miracle today, and from the bottom of my heart I want that for you. Work for your soul, your family, and for God. All things can be healed; remember that and believe.

Stop by our Itty Bitty™ website to find interesting information regarding healing and optimal health

www.IttyBittyPublishing.com

Or visit Angela Kung at:

www.angelakungacupuncture.com

www.theangelakung.com

@angela.kung.inspire

@angelakungacupuncture

Table of Contents

Introduction

Welcome to an Itty Bitty book containing a world of information. There is so much to say about how true healing works that it's impossible to touch upon all the subjects or dive deep enough into any that would answer all your questions. However, I'm deeply grateful that you are here and that you're reading this book to learn about how you can truly heal or help a loved one.

You, along with many others, have become more aware of the limits of conventional medicine and would like to understand more about energy healing and how it can change your life. Your destiny is not a life of chronic health problems or living with mental or emotional suffering. While healing is a challenging journey, it brings many rewards. It is the hardest and best thing you can accomplish for your soul's purpose and its work.

I wish you courage, faith, and many blessings on your journey to health and balance.

Because this book is about spirituality, I use the word God. If this offends you in any way, I ask that you replace the word God with any word you choose that represents your higher power.

Thank you, God bless you, and into the rabbit hole we go ...

Step 1
Health is a Spiritual Journey

Do you want to achieve good health mentally, emotionally, and physically? If so, then you should know that health is a spiritual journey. You came to this planet as a spirit, and spirit is at the heart of your healing and soul growth. You came to the earth plane to overcome obstacles and learn lessons so that your spirit could grow and earn the spiritual Ph.D. of life.

Some things you should know:

1. Your soul is pure consciousness, infinite, and full of light.
2. Your physical body is the temple of your soul.
3. Your physical body allows you to feel, hear, see, think, and experience life.
4. You are a divine spirit child of the infinite creator.
5. When your soul is happy and full of light, your mind and body thrive with vibrancy and good health.
6. When your soul is unhappy and experiences suffering or trauma, your mind and body weaken, becoming imbalanced, sick, and diseased.

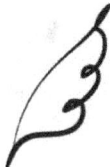

More About Health is a Spiritual Journey

Because illness can be mental, emotional, and physical, it's imperative to look at the spirit for the root cause. For instance, when we develop cancer, we must look deeper for the original trauma that started the imbalance to unwind and truly heal. This is why true healing is a spiritual journey.

Here are some examples of possible root causes of the dis-eases listed below:

- Physical, emotional, or sexual abuse may cause hypothyroidism and depression.
- Abandonment or lack of parental support may cause Crohn's disease and IBS.
- Parental divorce during childhood may cause unhealthy relationships, migraines, allergies, and obesity.
- Growing up with an addicted parent may cause codependency and unhealthy relationships.
- Being bullied at school may cause eating disorders, panic attacks, and low self-esteem.
- Frequent moving and changing schools in childhood may later cause anxiety or difficulty with social bonding.

Think of the ailments you suffer from and look forward to the spiritual lessons you came here to learn as you work through them. Healing is a journey of self-love, and love is medicine.

Step 2
Your Diagnosis Isn't Who You Are

Have you ever received a diagnosis that was overwhelming and made you feel hopeless? A diagnosis is not a proclamation, nor should it become part of your identity. It is merely a name for an ailment you may be experiencing, and ailments can be healed even if you have a well-known chronic disease. Remain unattached to the diagnosis and use the information wisely to begin seeking deeper answers for the root cause of your ailment.

Consider natural health methods such as:

1. Acupuncture and Chinese medicine
2. Energy medicine or energy healing
3. Reiki (in person or remote)
4. Craniosacral therapy
5. Spiritual healing methods (such as emotion code, body code, and theta healing)
6. Spiritual counseling

Many practitioners in these fields can help you discover more about yourself and what's beneath the surface.

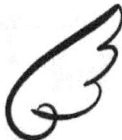

More About Your Diagnosis Isn't Who You Are

Since you are not the label of your diagnosis, let's first realize who you truly are:

- A light being
- A precious soul
- A child of God
- Pure divine love
- A spirit full of gifts and talents
- A spirit being, unconditionally loved and supported by your Creator

Your medical diagnosis should be a stepping-stone to inspire deeper healing, soul growth, learning, and more balance in your life. See your diagnosis as:

- A clue that deeper healing answers are waiting to be discovered to improve your life.
- Practical information to provide a compass for you on your spiritual path.
- Inspiration to help you find spiritual meaning.
- A chance to heal and grow spiritually.
- A rewarding test of faith during the healing process.
- A journey of self-love and compassion.
- A relationship builder with God.

Step 3
Spiritual Dis-Ease Manifests as Physical Disease

Your body is your temple, your best friend, and a divine gift from God. It has been your servant, doing what you've asked it to do all these years. And when it stops working well, you blame it. But your body was just doing what you told it to do. The issue began in your spirit long before it manifested in the body.

1. Your spirit became imbalanced first.
2. Your mind and emotional well-being began to suffer the consequences.
3. Finally, your physical body got sick and developed chronic pain or even cancer.

By the time your body has symptoms, it could be 40 years before a deadly disease develops.

1. Be aware of your mental and emotional pains.
2. Realize the importance of healing your pains.
3. Prevent physical disease by healing the mental, emotional, and spiritual bodies.
4. The idea of "being strong" and "sweeping problems under the rug" is dangerous.

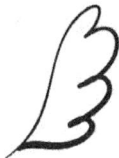

5

More About Spiritual Dis-Ease Manifests as Physical Disease

Here are more examples of spiritual dis-eases manifesting as physical diseases (see Step 1):

- Migraines may be rooted in a verbally abusive childhood.
- Irritable bowel syndrome may be rooted in parental abandonment.
- Cancer can be rooted in unworthiness from childhood molestation and shame.
- Seizures and ADHD may be rooted in the mother's traumatic stress during pregnancy.
- Bipolar disorder may be rooted in sexual trauma during childhood.
- Fibromyalgia may stem from growing up in a toxic family environment.
- Parasites or mold toxicity may be rooted in abuse and lack of support in youth.
- High blood pressure from growing up during wartime or a drama-filled home.
- Low back pain from workaholism rooted in self-abuse, self-sabotage, and unfor-giveness after abuse from parents during childhood.

Every experience has a consequence, but the good news is that you can heal the original trauma and change the results of how it impacts your life.

Step 4
The Traumas You Experience Affect Your Health and Balance

Most people do not believe that trauma affects their health. That's because your survival mechanism automatically protects you by storing trauma until you can consciously work through the gravity and sometimes the shock of it. Imagine running away from a bear and getting a splinter in the process. Pulling out that splinter will have to wait!

The problem with the survival mechanism is:

1. Trauma energy still lives in you.
2. Trauma may continue to steal energy from you, wearing down your health.
3. You repeat the same trauma with different players or experiences until the original trauma is pulled out or healed.

This is not well understood because most people will downplay their trauma or say they never had trauma in their past. Yes, your protective mechanism is that strong!

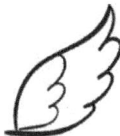

More About How Trauma Affects Your Health

Why do we bury trauma or refuse to deal with it?

- It's too painful to bring up.
- You're afraid no one will understand.
- You don't want to be vulnerable.
- You think it will just go away if unspoken, so why cause more trouble?
- You don't think healing is possible.
- Your pride gets in the way.

Here are common symptoms that occur when you bury trauma:

- Physical health issues
- Feeling of heaviness
- Anxiety
- Panic attacks
- Depression
- Chronic fatigue
- Fibromyalgia
- Failed relationships
- Anger, resentment, emotional illness
- Mental illness/loneliness
- Suicidal thoughts
- Repetitive negative and harmful patterns
- Cysts, tumors, and cancer
- Autoimmune diseases
- ADD, ADHD, bipolar disorder, OCD
- Addictions

Step 5
Emotions and Belief Systems Make or Break Your Health

Negative emotions and belief systems come from trauma, negative experiences, and are even absorbed from our parents or environment. In fact, they can even be inherited from the energy in the DNA passed down to you. Here are some examples of negative belief systems:

1. I'm a loser who is always picked on.
2. I don't have a good relationship with money; I'll always struggle.
3. I'm just like my mom, I'm not marriage material for men.
4. Women can't be trusted; they just want you for your money.
5. Telling your children they're stupid makes them work harder.
6. Saying *I love you* is a sign of weakness.
7. Truly loving someone isn't safe.
8. Marriage is just a financial contract.
9. I can't be my true self because no one will like me.
10. I'm not loveable, so I'll always be alone.
11. I'll never be good enough.
12. I'm not smart, so I have to use my looks to get by.

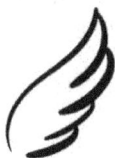

More About How Emotions and Belief Systems Make or Break Your Health

Thoughts with negative emotional charges bring a frequency into your body that increases tension, inflammation, acidity, pain, stress, nerve damage, hormonal imbalance, and brain disorders. Furthermore, they can negatively affect your cells, tissues, tendons, ligaments, muscles, vessels, and organs.

Here's what you can do to get on a healing path. Find a practitioner who can intuitively help you:

- Garner the courage to do the work.
- Dig deeper to find and heal the original trauma.
- Work to clear negative emotional frequencies.
- Cut unhealthy energy cording.
- Release evil energies occupying your body and energy field.
- Clear blockages in the body's energy meridians and balance chakras.
- Clear generational traumas, curses, and belief systems.
- Remove unforgiveness and resentment.
- Download positive frequencies and beliefs needed to heal.
- Do the inner child work to become whole and connected again.

Step 6
Anxiety and Depression Lead the Way

Are you struggling with anxiety and depression? Instead of seeing anxiety, panic, bipolar disorder, depression, or even suicidal depression as a negative, shameful thing, you need to see these ailments as powerful indicators leading the way to the root of your problem. These ailments are actually key ways or necessary symptoms that your mind, body, and spirit use to communicate with you, letting you know that something is wrong.

Anxiety, depression, or other mood disorders are:

1. Ways the mind, body, and spirit communicate that something is deeply wrong and needs attention.
2. Key indicators during the healing process to know whether more healing is needed.
3. Important symptoms to be grateful for.

It's time to remove the fear of judgment and begin doing the work of self-love and healing.

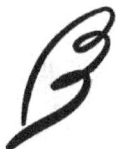

More About Anxiety and Depression Leading the Way

If you have been suffering emotionally or mentally, reach out for help, and don't give up on yourself. You are worth it! The rewards for working through the tough healing process are great. Talk to those who have the ability to understand or listen with compassion about your feelings and strive to seek the right professional help.

Here are some professionals to consider:

- Psychologist
- Social worker
- Psychiatrist (meds may be necessary, at least at the beginning of your journey)

A holistic wellness professional who specializes in psycho-emotional disorders and trauma-related issues is ideal, including some of the following:

- Acupuncturist
- Chinese herbalist
- Energy healer
- Spiritual healer
- Spiritual counselor
- Theta healer
- Emotion code/body code healer
- Reiki master
- Craniosacral therapist
- Massage therapist

Step 7
Soul Opposition and Distraction

Planet Earth is a world of opposition and opposites. There's up and down, left and right, man and woman, hot and cold. There's also good and evil. In Chinese medicine, the acupuncturist or Qi Gong energy healer works to eliminate evil energy while tonifying righteous qi. In some religious faiths, there are evil entities and demons to contend with. To understand health, you must understand that your body is a container for your soul; it can host light or it can host darkness. It can host love or it can host hate energy. If your soul is pure conscious light energy, and you live in a world of opposition, doesn't it make sense that there must be oppositional energy against your light?

1. Your soul is made of pure light energy.
2. The opposing force aims to steal your light energy and increase darkness.
3. Knowing this and knowing that your goal is to defend your light and remove darkness is key to healing.
4. Trauma is a major cause of darkness.
5. Negative emotions and belief systems perpetuate dark energy.

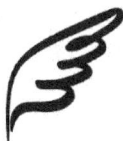

More About Soul Opposition and Distraction

Distractions are opposing forces to deceive your receipt of truth and love. They block you from seeing clearly, like a fog that leads you away from true healing. Some things seem good, but underneath the surface, they distract you from healing.

Some examples of distractions:

- Addiction to drugs, alcohol, coffee, school, work, sex, food, and shopping
- Excessive entertainment such as video games, sports, TV, and social media
- Toxic relationships in marriage, dating, and friendship

Other less obvious distractions:

- Cultural demands, such as a career choice made to please your parents
- High-adrenaline activities
- Competition, money, or power mis-aligned with your highest good or your soul purpose

Most things have two sides like a coin. Your job is to honestly evaluate the things in your life that serve a higher purpose, or distractions that detract from your soul's growth, learning, and healing.

Step 8
Relationships Affect Your Health: Love Should Be a Win-Win

Relationships can be detrimental to your health mentally, emotionally, physically, and spiritually. Some are abusive and toxic. Decide what you need to heal or learn from relationships to begin the task of healing. Evaluate the relationships in your life to see if they need improvement and to discover what you believe about yourself.

1. How the other person treats you says a lot about what you think you deserve.
2. The other person only triggers things you must contend with. Thank them for it.
3. Generational patterns or belief systems may need to be cleared to change things.
4. Trauma may need to be cleared to shift negative energy to positive energy.

Adopt an attitude of gratitude for recognizing where you need to focus attention.

1. The other person is here to play a role you need to change, heal, and grow. Forgive them and give thanks.
2. Your spirit came to earth to overcome this so you become wiser for it.

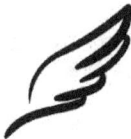

More About Making Relationships a Win-Win Deal

Earth is our spirit school and relationships are very often our classrooms. All relationships are learning grounds for healing, growth, and love.

How do you create win-win relationships?

- Work through the trauma that relationships trigger to clear negative emotions and resentment.
- Know that God loves you unconditionally; let your guard down to receive it.
- Learn to love yourself unconditionally as well; nourish your inner child.
- See the other person as a victim of their own trauma and pain to know it's not about you.
- Love and accept the other person without judgment.
- Apply healthy boundaries with the other person, even if they don't like it at first.
- Show them a healthy version of you and your love for them.

Congratulations! By doing the above you are stronger for healing through your own pain and creating an opportunity for the other person to come into their own light as well. It's a win-win.

All divine relationships are mutually beneficial.

Step 9
Codependency: The Old Way of Love

Look around you and you'll find that more than half the people you know have unhealthy relationships wrought with codependent ties. You should never be "tied" to anyone—the very word relays being "stuck" or "handcuffed."

1. You might believe that codependent relationships are the definition of love.
2. You may not realize that you have codependent relationships.
3. Your codependent nature may be the result of your upbringing and what you know of relationship love.

You are codependent if you:

1. Go beyond healthy boundaries to help or save others.
2. Lose yourself in relationships and feel toxic, exhausted, anxious, or depressed.
3. Find yourself in relationships with addicts and narcissists.

You can heal by clearing past (even ancestral) traumas, curses, and spells, as well as your own traumas of unworthiness and fear.

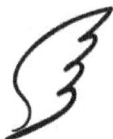

More About Codependency: The Old Way of Love

Here's a way to picture a codependent relationship: think of a loved one stuck in a ditch screaming for help. You jump right in and now both of you are stuck. Since relationships should be win-win, you'd be better off finding a ladder to let them climb out on their own.

- The person in the ditch may decide to climb out now, later, or never. Respect the decision they make.
- Detach yourself from their emotional pull and let them work through their pain.
- Discover healthy ways to support them that doesn't drain your energy.
- Be prepared for them to throw a tantrum.
- You suffer/feel resentment when you try to help or save them. This enables and disables them.
- Your codependency will heal as you back away with healthier boundaries.
- Use your free agency to save yourself; focus on healing you.

The metaphorical ladder can be:

- A hug, a loving letter, supportive words.
- A kind gesture to show you care.
- Giving responsibility back so they are accountable and thus empowered.
- Making healthy choices that positively influence them to do the same.

Step 10
Emotional Freedom is
the Key to Good Health

Emotional freedom is the foundation of good health. You must let go of your negative emotions and resentments, as well as those of others you've absorbed to give your cells the vibrant frequency they need to thrive.

Find a healer who can help you to:

1. Clear negative emotions and unforgiveness at the deepest levels.
2. Clear traumatic memories that keep your cells unhealthy and your nervous system in fight or flight.
3. Clear trauma from before you entered the womb, time in the womb, and your exit (birth).
4. Clear all negative energies on the ancestral, soul, and DNA levels.
5. Cleanse and heal your energy field to help you shift into a healthier you.
6. Clear negative and evil entities in your space, mind, body, home, and workspace.
7. Cut unhealthy attachments in unhealthy relationships.
8. Remove negative repetitive patterns.

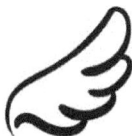

More About Emotional Freedom as the Key to Good Health

Sometimes you don't know what your emotional issues are—you just know you don't feel great. If you just bring those issues or "blocks" to your healing sessions, your energy or spiritual healer can help you uncover the roots. It's both a process and a journey, so be patient with yourself. All truths will be revealed in due time, and all things will heal in divine timing.

What can you do to achieve emotional freedom?

- Recognize when you utilize distractions to avoid feelings such as toxic relationships or addictions, and also sports, eating disorders, etc.
- Find a health professional to talk to when difficult feelings arise.
- Work toward relieving root causes.
- Try the EFT tapping technique.
- Find a psychiatrist for medication as a temporary option if needed.
- Get bodywork like acupuncture, massage, etc., (see Step 2).

Unhealthy emotions block your energy pathways and affect your brain and moods. Working on healing them and finding emotional freedom is the spiritual work you came to do. You'll have more joy, peace, and vibrant health!

Step 11
The Dead Are Here to Help

Have you experienced a deceased loved one coming to your aid or trying to communicate with you? Often, your deceased ancestors are the ones guiding you along your spiritual path. They are the angels in your life.

1. Your deceased ancestors, friends, or relatives can help guide and support you.
2. As you pray or meditate, try communicating with them as well.
3. All unfinished business with your loved ones can still be healed.

You may be sensitive to a loved one's energy around you, communicating and receiving love and guidance. Seek out a spiritual healer who has intuitive abilities to help in this process.

1. True health comes from consciously living a spiritual life.
2. Know that we are all spirits; we don't disappear when we die. Knowing this removes the fear of death.
3. Fear of death and not understanding your spiritual nature negatively impacts your health.

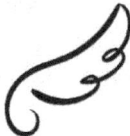

More About the Dead Are Here to Help

So much grief, shock, and trauma occur when loved ones pass on. You should know that you can heal from these emotions and can even heal unfinished business after their mortal life.

Work with a spiritual energy healer to:

- Clear the shock, trauma, and grief from the passing of a loved one.
- Clear and resolve unfinished business, negative emotions, unhealthy attachments, or traumas with a loved one.
- Help your loved one communicate with you or help them with something they need.

There are instances when a loved one might be stuck (earthbound) and needs assistance to cross over. They may simply need to say something to you. Their human ego is gone, and they more clearly see the spiritual truths of the bigger divine picture. Therefore, they can love you and accept you when perhaps they couldn't during their human life.

- Be aware of the support and spirit guidance that is available to you.
- Release residual anger and fear.
- Connect spiritually and embrace them.
- Let love flow through you and enjoy blessings from your loved ones.

Step 12
Believing You Can Heal
Makes All the Difference

When a medical doctor gives a patient a death
sentence, such as four weeks to live, most likely,
they will die in exactly four weeks. What about
patients who go on living and eventually heal?
They didn't believe they would die as predicted.
They *believed* they would live.

1. Believe you can heal, and you will.
2. You don't always need to know how you
   will heal; just believe, and have faith.
3. Ask and seek the next breadcrumb, and it
   will appear.
4. You must *want* to heal for it to happen
   and take the necessary actions.

If you believe you can heal but don't *want* to
heal, that's a major problem. If you're in this
category, there are likely deep unresolved
traumas that have been there a long time. You
must work extra hard to save your own life and
work through troubled thoughts and emotions.
Seek a professional energy worker, light worker,
or spiritual healer to help you navigate out of the
darkness. You may also seek out a therapist,
social worker, or temporary medication from a
psychiatrist for extra support.

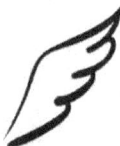

More About Believing You Can Heal Makes All the Difference

If you believe you can heal, and it is in God's will for you to stay on earth longer, your spirit will align with the process of your healing.

- Your spirit aligns and draws experiences to help you heal.
- Your brain sends the right signals to your body.
- Your hormones, mood, and outlook shift your frequency for health and vitality.

Believing is the first step to healing. Here are additional steps:

- Find your *why*—your higher purpose.
- Clear the deep traumas and blocks to self-love and self-resentment.
- Forgive God and others in your life.
- Accept the lessons you must overcome.
- Understand that life issues don't just go away when your body dies.
- Commit to yourself that you are your number one priority.
- Know that whatever seems impossible is possible with God.

Living a human life is a gift we're given, despite its hardships. You chose to come into this life to learn the tough lessons that grow your spirit to become more like God.

Step 13
How Self-Reliance and Self-Empowerment Bring Health

Have you ever heard the following statement: "We come into this world alone, and we leave it alone?" No one can do those things for you, and no one can live your life for you. Your job is to learn self-reliance in this life to become self-empowered. God is there for you, but you must do the work.

1. Accept the responsibility of living your own life and stop depending on others for things you can do yourself.
2. Take responsibility for yourself to increase confidence, which enables you to take charge of your own health.
3. Keep healthy boundaries so others can have self-reliance too, which is important to your health and their health. Remember to stay in your own lane.
4. Have patience to learn the things you struggle with to grow your faith in God who will empower you.
5. Love yourself enough to know that you can do anything you put your mind to.

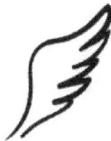

More About How Self-Reliance and Self-Empowerment Bring Health

In order to thrive in your life, you must have an "I can do it" attitude. Know that you are supported by the spiritual network of love that you typically can't see: God, angels, spirit guides, deceased loved ones, plus the living.

- Do at least one thing a day that empowers you.
- Set goals for yourself and take the necessary steps to achieve them.
- Rely on yourself to figure things out as much as possible.
- Ask for help and seek guidance to learn things to do for yourself.
- You are not meant to do everything yourself, which is why we have families, friends, communities, and the divine order to help you.

Self-reliance is an important divine concept. If you understand how this helps in your spiritual journey, you can improve the health of your mind, body, and spirit. Self-reliance increases your:

- Confidence
- Peace and joy
- Life experience as rewarding
- Empathy and compassion
- Spiritual wisdom

Step 14
Claim Your Power, Claim Your Gifts

You came into this world with natural talents and gifts. Some need to be honed and some are accessible right away. Here are some examples:

1. You have a musical gift to play the guitar without ever taking lessons.
2. You excel in mathematics, which comes to you easily; you innately understand it.
3. You dance with grace and move to music naturally in ways that reveal your gift of movement.
4. You love to build. Creating blueprints for ultra-luxurious resorts is challenging, fun, and yet, easy for you.

To claim your power to achieve greater health:

1. Claim the gifts you've been given by using them to serve God and serve others.
2. Respect your gifts, God, and yourself by using them for the greater good.
3. Use your divine gifts to empower people to increase light, love, and health to the whole world.
4. Stand tall in your gifts and if they are taken from you, work to reclaim them.

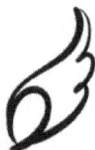

More About Claim Your Power, Claim Your Gifts

You might not realize that there are other gifts you can be born with. Let's call them gifts of the spirit.

Here are some examples of gifts of the spirit:

- You know when someone in your family just died or is going to die.
- You communicate with animals.
- You know how others are feeling without being told.
- You have a knowing of things that logically you shouldn't know.
- You see spirits and feel their energy.
- You can communicate with those who have passed through hearing, seeing, feeling, smelling, or knowing.

To claim your power and live your best life, don't be afraid of your gifts; thank God for them and use them for the higher good of all.

- Love and develop your gifts.
- Learn to use your gifts with excellence.
- Help yourself and others thrive by using your gifts for good.
- Empower yourself and your vibrancy of life with your gifts.

Step 15
Preparing for the Beautiful Transition
Called Death

When you know that you have a finite amount of
time to live there are many things to do: overcome obstacles, learn spiritual lessons, heal
yourself and your relationships, claim and hone
your gifts to excellence, attain knowledge and
wisdom you came to learn, and live out a pur-
pose-filled life. You can consciously prepare for
the wonderful passage of going home, commonly
known as "death," which strengthens your vitality
and health while on this earth.

1. Remove your fear of death.
2. See your earthly life as an opportunity to
   heal, love, learn, and grow while having
   fun and experiencing joy.
3. Accept the work set out for you in life
   and reap the rewards for doing it.
4. Life is like a video game with endless
   lives. Every day you get to try again.
5. Be conscious about soul work that needs
   healing and apply yourself.
6. Prepare for the passage home with
   confidence that you've covered all bases.

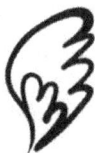

More About Preparing for the Beautiful Transition Called Death

If you are ready to die or know that it is coming, you can still accomplish a lot of healing before you cross over.

Work with a professional healer to help you:

- Release lingering trauma and resentment.
- Clear regrets.
- Ask God for forgiveness.
- Forgive yourself and forgive others.
- Connect to your inner child.
- Communicate with God and those on the other side.

It takes courage to do the soul work you came to do to live your best life with good health.

- Don't give up; have patience.
- Healing is not a straight line.
- You were born into a body with existing generational problems.
- If there's a will, there's a way.
- Change repetitive negative patterns.
- Nourish and heal your soul every day.
- Shine your light on others; it feeds you.
- Do the healing work to prepare yourself.
- Live consciously for the finish line.
- Go home happy and satisfied!

You've finished. Before you go ...

Post/Share that you finished this book.

Please star-rate this book.

Reviews are solid gold to writers. Please take a few minutes to give us some itty bitty feedback.

ABOUT THE AUTHOR

Angela Kung is the CEO of Angela Kung Acupuncture & Wellness Center in Mission Viejo,
CA. As a young child, she was highly sensitive to
energy and intuition. She had the gift of knowing
and healing. At the age of six, she informed her
parents that she would grow up to be a doctor.

She discovered ice skating, fell in love with it,
and pursued competitive skating and coaching.
Along the way in her life, Angela faced
emotional trauma, injuries, and health challenges,
which ultimately sparked her intuitive healing
abilities and a passion for helping herself and
others.

When conventional medicine didn't help and
Angela felt anxious, lost, depressed, and in
chronic pain, she decided against medical school.
Her healing journey took her into the world of
energy and spiritual healing, which would change
her life. She honed her gifts and passionately
began to help others. Angela now works as a:
Spiritual counselor, Energy healer, Lightworker,
Acupuncturist, Chinese herbalist, Theta healer,
Reiki master, Author, Educator, and Speaker.

Her expertise in healing spiritual dis-ease
includes: Psycho-emotional disorders,
Generational and inherited diseases, Relationship
issues, Internal medicine diseases and Autoimmune diseases, Neuropathic diseases, Cancer,
and Rare diseases from over 25 years of real-life
experience and patient cases.

Her affinity for miracles began when she needed them herself, and after experiencing so many in her life, they are now a part of the everyday experience when she works with her patients.

Angela understands that true healing often takes place outside the box of conventional medicine. She takes her patients on incredible healing journeys to the soul's core, allowing the mind, emotional body, and physical body to follow.

Her mission is to help as many people as possible to truly heal. She gathers the most gifted, loving healing professionals at her wellness center to compassionately care for those in need. She invites you to her sacred healing space where you will become enlightened, healed, and changed for the better.

Angela grew up in Massachusetts until her spiritual calling took her to California, where she finished school and opened her practice in 2010. She resides in Mission Viejo with her husband and continues to ice skate, because dancing on ice ignites her heart and soul!

Angela won the title of 2025 Mrs. Asia USA of Virgelia Productions and attributes this honor to being part of her spiritual calling and pathway to her growth and success as a healer and inspiration for others.

www.angelakungacupuncture.com

If you enjoyed this Itty Bitty™ book, you might also like…

- **Your Amazing Itty Bitty™ Spirituality Book** ~ Rev. Summer Albayati

- **Your Amazing Itty Bitty™ Relationships as a Spiritual Practice** ~ Deborah A. Gayle

- **Your Amazing Itty Bitty™ Grief Book** ~ Lisa Y. Herrington

Or any of the many other Amazing Itty Bitty™ books available online at
www.ittybittypublishing.com

www.ingramcontent.com/pod-product-compliance
Lightning Source LLC
Chambersburg PA
CBHW060659280326
41933CB00012B/2248